WHAT YOU SHOULD KNOW ABOUT SLEEP APNEA

AN EASY TO UNDERSTAND GUIDE

Other Books by Dr. Nicholas DiFilippo

What You Should Know About Asthma and Other Lung Diseases: Essential Information for Patients and Families

Recognizing Symptoms of Common Lung Diseases: Causes and Treatment of Shortness of Breath, Cough, and Chest Pain

The Ventilator Dependent Patient: End of Life Issue? A Pulmonologist's Perspective

To Munich Rome and Back Home: Lessons from Travel to Germany, Austria and Italy

ALL AVAILABLE AS PRINT AND KINDLE EDITIONS

WHAT YOU SHOULD KNOW ABOUT SLEEP APNEA

AN EASY TO UDERSTAND GUIDE

———

DR. NICHOLAS DIFILIPPO
PULMONOLOGIST

WHAT YOU SHOULD KNOW ABOUT SLEEP APNEA
Copyright © 2013 by NICHOLAS DIFILIPPO, INTERNAL MEDICINE AND PULMONARY DISEASES

All rights reserved. No part of this book may be reproduced or transmitted in any form or by any means without written permission from the author.

ISBN-13: 978-1482025156
ISBN-10: 1482025159

Printed in USA

Dedication

This book, like my prior books, is dedicated to all my former patients. My patients were the foundation for my previous books and they also remain the foundation for this current book. All my patients have given me a precious gift, the wonderful opportunity to study and practice my first love, pulmonary medicine. Each patient brought his own unique perspective to whatever disease process was unfolding. I have never been one to endorse a cookie-cutter approach to patient care. Certain principles of medicine apply to each disease, but not necessarily to the individual patient. Patient care and personal relationships transcend these principles. Patients are much more than a collection of diseases or puzzles of symptoms to be solved. Patients actually become an integral part of all of us that have had the privilege of practicing medicine and serving patients and their families.

Table of Contents

Dedication 5

Table of Contents 6

Preface 7

Acknowledgments 9

Introduction to this Series 11

Chapter 1: INTRODUCTION TO SLEEP APNEA 15

Chapter 2: MEDICAL FACTS YOU SHOULD KNOW ABOUT SLEEP APNEA 19

Chapter 3: DISEASES WITH SIMILARITY TO SLEEP APNEA 41

Chapter 4: FACTS YOU SHOULD KNOW ABOUT THE MEDICAL TREATMENT OF SLEEP APNEA 45

Chapter 5: WHAT DOES ALL THIS MEAN FOR YOU? 51

Chapter 6: SUMMARY 55

Questions 57

Answers and Discussion 61

INDEX 67

About the Author 69

Preface

Pulmonary medicine is an exciting and intellectually challenging field of medicine. For the uninitiated, pulmonary medicine concerns treatment of patients with lung diseases. A physician practicing pulmonary medicine is known as a pulmonologist. Not too many people are familiar with this term, but almost everyone is familiar with a cardiologist. A cardiologist, as you most likely know, treats patients with heart diseases; a pulmonologist works next door with the lungs and treats patients with lung diseases. A pulmonologist deals with diseases such as emphysema, bronchitis, pulmonary fibrosis, hypersensitivity pneumonitis, as well as numerous lesser known diseases. Each disease presents its own rather unique set of medical facts. Sleep apnea, a lung disease, is no exception. Sleep apnea is a captivating and very active field of study. Much research is going on in this field and many diverse disciplines, other than pulmonary medicine, are involved in its study. This book is meant to introduce and inform you, the reader, about various important medical aspects related to this disease. Let it be your guide. As is true of practically every disease, medical aspects of a disease take true meaning only when the patient is viewed and treated as the unique, important human being that he truly is. Moreover, sleep apnea can leave its imprint on human behavior and human interaction. It can affect many aspects of daily living.

After having practiced pulmonary medicine, in a hospital and office setting, for several decades, I am well aware that time spent in a physician's office is frequently short. There is a schedule to maintain and many issues to be covered. This often results in too little time for a complete discussion of all the issues. The hospital setting, on the other hand, may provide some increased time for interaction, but usually so many activities are taking place at the same time that patients often have rather vague recollections of any pertinent discussions that did take place. This book is meant to enhance medical knowledge and allow more productive interaction between physicians, patients and family members. Think of it as a possible extension of physician time. It is also meant to help you realize and consider the possibility of sleep apnea as a cause of some difficulties during activities of daily living. A clear and fairly comprehensive discussion of sleep apnea, its various medical correlations, and its relationship to activities of daily living are presented in the following pages.

This book, like every other medically related book, can never be considered to be specific advice for any one individual. Medical books explain general medical principles that can be applied in certain diseases, but only in a very general and nonspecific way. By necessity the explanations are only of a general nature. Never assume that any specific principle necessarily applies to you. Therefore, this book, like all other medical books, can only provide a supplement to personal physician advice and knowledge. No specificity to any reader or individual is intended or implied by any statement.

Acknowledgments

I wish to acknowledge the fine work of individuals who have helped to make this book a reality. The excellent cover design represents the hard work of Nicholas Liesen. The technical ideas for this book represent the much appreciated input of Christopher Liesen. I also wish to acknowledge the encouragement and support of my lifelong friend and periodontist, Dr. Larry Jenkins, without whom this book would never have come to fruition. I would be remiss not to acknowledge the input of my family both to this book and to my life in general. Often, throughout the years, they found themselves playing "second fiddle" to my pursuit of pulmonary medicine. I also wish to acknowledge the impetus given me by Gregory McGovern in initiating this project.

Introduction to this Series

Sleep apnea should be as familiar and as well known by the general public as common diseases such as emphysema, Alzheimer's disease, or heart attack. Sleep apnea is much more common than you may think. Its manifestations are widespread. It affects routine every day activity in many ways. Awareness of its existence is essential. This is because the disease is often insidious and may be present for many years before its existence is even suspected. If one does not know about the disease or about what effects it may have on human life, it will never be discovered or even thought of during its early stages. As you will see throughout this book, sleep apnea can easily affect your life without you even knowing it. That problem that may be annoying you may not be because you're growing old. The problem may not be that you are forgetful or that you are easily distracted. You might not simply be sleepy. These issues may have a root cause. The problem may actually be sleep apnea. Manifestations of sleep apnea may have many other causes, and often these other causes come to mind rather than the possibility of sleep apnea.

One of the primary purposes of this book is to increase awareness of sleep apnea. Often patients go around for years having a little bit of difficulty here and a little bit of difficulty there and not really thinking much about what the real problem may be. Changes, being gradual, often go completely unnoticed or they may be ignored and "placed on the back burner." A person may wake up with a morning headache, take some medication and then forget about the problem. He may be told that he snores a lot during sleep and he may even notice that he does not feel refreshed in the morning. He might just shrug his shoulders and subsequently downplay these observations. Neither he nor the person making comments about his sleep may consider any other realistic possibility as to cause. Many hints may be dropped and ignored along the way, but if someone does not think about the possibility of sleep apnea, evaluation will be delayed and problems may gradually worsen. If you are not aware of the possibility of subtle changes early in the course of sleep apnea, how can you do something about it? Either you or someone who sees you in action has to be cognizant of the possibility. The topic of sleep apnea is not just about a lung disease, it is actually about human life in general. As one of my college professors used to say just before making an important point, "Listen with both ears in high gear." In this case, however, also put your eyes and brain in high gear and enjoy the ride. Although a quick read, this little book should be a helpful, practical, and useful guide to sleep apnea. You will soon be surprised by what you have learned while reading this book, especially when you answer the questions towards the back of this book.

This text is based on my book *WHAT YOU SHOULD KNOW ABOUT ASTHMA AND OTHER LUNG DISEASES*. It is not simply a reproduction of a section of that book. Instead, it is an expanded consideration of one particular lung disorder, sleep apnea. It represents the first of a proposed series of *WHAT YOU SHOULD KNOW ABOUT ……. (some particular individual lung disease)*. *WHAT YOU SHOULD KNOW ABOUT SLEEP APNEA* consequently represents the first in this proposed series of publications. Each is meant to provide a detailed explanation of a particular ailment. The explanation should be understandable to all with a reasonable educational background. It is not meant for the professional medical provider. It is meant for you - the layman. The layman may thus be able to adequately understand the individual pulmonary disease. This should be helpful not only for better medical care but also for furthering overall understanding of various aspects of human existence and diseases. Additionally, the reader will be able to adequately discuss and intelligently ask questions regarding various aspects of a particular disease with his physician and consequently improve health care through better understanding of the issues involved in each disease. Please note that I am speaking about asking questions regarding a particular disease and related health issues, not questioning your physician. There is a definite distinction here. Knowledge, questioning and understanding go hand-in-hand. Knowledge is power. Medical care and lung diseases are no exception.

As noted in the *PREFACE* to this book, medical comments and principles necessarily pertain to any reader only in a general way. Any medically related book can offer only general knowledge regarding any topic. This book is no exception. Specificity can come only from a personal physician that has knowledge of all general medical principles and knowledge and specificity of any particular situation and individual.

Chapter 1: INTRODUCTION TO SLEEP APNEA

Consider the following potential situations: 1) You are waiting at a red light. Your friend is driving the car in front of you. The light changes, but the car in front of you does not begin to move until the green light is almost over and you politely tap on your horn. You are puzzled, what is going on - was my friend only distracted? 2) It is three o'clock in the afternoon and you are talking on the phone to your friend. You notice that the friend does not quite respond appropriately to the discussion. In fact, he may not respond at all. You have to yell into the phone in order to get his attention and appropriate response. Why is he acting like that? He is not hard of hearing. 3) It is a summer evening and you are walking down the street, enjoying the beautiful weather. You walk by your friend's house where the windows are open and the air conditioning is not on. You hear someone snoring loudly. You note that the breathing is irregular. You also hear what appears to be gasping and choking. There are what appear to be periods of silence with the absence of snoring. Why all those bizarre noises? 4) Your friend is returning from work and is involved in an auto accident. As a matter of fact he has had several minor accidents within the past year. Is this normal? 5) Your friend has elevated blood pressure that he says his physician finds difficult to control. He may complain of a morning headache, having gained weight recently and having difficulty in concentrating. He might appear to be somewhat drowsy during the daytime and a bit slow to respond. What accounts for this?

Remember the movies *ANALYZE THIS* and *ANALYZE THAT*? Well stop to analyze this: What do the above situations represent? Are these situations just the way things are with human behavior - what is to be expected as time marches on?

Is there any need for further concern and analysis? These everyday situations appear to be rather commonplace and innocuous. However, although commonplace they are not necessarily innocuous. There is a need to evaluate these situations further. Stop and consider the possibility that your friend may actually have sleep apnea. These types of scenarios may be some of the everyday experiences of patients with sleep apnea. The changes described may be so gradual that they often go unnoticed. Patients with sleep apnea may encounter numerous unexplained subtle difficulties as they go about their activities of daily life. They may need help from others in order for them to realize that something serious is going on. Over time, potential harm may occur because of the medical problem of sleep apnea. Hopefully, after reading this text, you will be familiar enough with the problem to discover it while it is still somewhat subtle. That is a goal of this text. If the problem is not realized by someone, no appropriate corrective action can ever be taken. However, by someone realizing the existence of a problem, potential harm may be averted. This might even be you. The person with sleep apnea can seek professional medical help in a timely fashion - well before serious harm may occur. As sleep apnea is quite common, knowledge about this interesting but serious disease should be helpful to any of us who have encountered situations similar to those enumerated above. These situations are all too common. If you have not encountered similar situations yet, either they were too subtle to be noted or you will soon encounter these types of situations. These situations may, in the appropriate context, represent sleep apnea. However, they might not. They may present in a similar fashion but the reason for their occurrence may be other than sleep apnea. How do you tell the difference? Read on and hopefully we can understand the underlying causes. As our story unfolds, it will take us into classical literature as well as into somewhat complex medical issues. You may understand classical literature, but fear understanding of complex medical issues. Fear not. The complex medical issues will be explained with clarity in detail and thereby be made understandable to all readers, regardless of their medical background.

    Before jumping directly into our topic of sleep apnea, we will need to have some understanding of sleep. Sleep is not a static state where you just lie there until you awaken. A number of activities take place during so-called quiet restful sleep. Under the right circumstances, some of these activities may predispose to adverse events. Basically, sleep can be divided into two major states. One is known as non-rapid eye movement (non-REM) sleep and the other as rapid eye movement (REM) sleep. Non-REM sleep is considered to be quiet sleep while REM sleep is considered to be active. Non-REM sleep, or quiet sleep, is further divided into stages, depending on the depth of sleep. The deepest sleep occurs in stage 4 and the lightest in stage 1. Sometimes the stages of sleep are classified as only being stage 1 to stage 3, with stage 3 being the deepest stage. At any rate, whatever staging is used, the deepest stages show what is called slow wave sleep. Dreams occur during REM sleep. Naturally, during REM sleep the brain is stimulated intensely. Remember, it is in REM sleep that rapid eye movements occur and dreams take place. Hence this state of sleep is designated as the active state of sleep. Normally, non-REM sleep and REM sleep alternate in an orderly fashion throughout the night. The active state of sleep alternates in a predictable way with the quiet state of sleep. Consequently, REM sleep may last 10 to 20 minutes and recur every 90 to 120 minutes. In between, non-REM sleep occurs. These time periods change somewhat as we progress from infancy to old age. The overall breathing pattern is affected slightly by both the state of sleep (REM or non-REM sleep) and stage of sleep (stage 1 to stage 4). In healthy individuals, the state or stage of sleep has, at most, only minimal effect on the breathing pattern. In medically unstable individuals, however, the breathing pattern may be predisposed to disruption.

Chapter 2: MEDICAL FACTS YOU SHOULD KNOW ABOUT SLEEP APNEA

The term "apnea" refers to lack of breathing. An apnea monitor thus monitors one's breathing, or lack of it. When combined with the term "sleep," the reference is to lack of breathing during sleep. Consequently, this type of disorder falls under the broad heading of sleep related breathing disorders. The field of sleep medicine is a very active field currently, and much research is being done in this field by a number of disciplines. New information is constantly being uncovered. Sleep medicine physicians, pulmonologists, neurologists, ENT, and also dentists are some of the disciplines studying the field of sleep apnea. The field of sleep medicine is also a field that borrows heavily from both history and classical literature. Unusual and captivating terms encountered in this field include "Pickwickian syndrome" and "Ondine's curse." We will explore these terms from the literature and relate them to problems concerning sleep related breathing disorders as this section unfolds. You will see the formation of alchemy - a marriage - of literature and medicine in this intriguing and captivating field of medicine. A vibrant area of medicine will thus unfold before your very eyes.

Trouble with breathing in patients with sleep apnea may be the result of either difficulty with initiating the respiratory cycle or difficulty with mechanical interference with the breathing cycle. Additionally it may be a mixed disorder containing elements of both. These two problems are referred to as central sleep apnea and obstructive sleep apnea. This division represents an important distinction as the causes and treatments of these two groups are vastly different. The central type of sleep apnea is much less common than the other, the obstructive sleep apnea. It is believed that central sleep apnea occurs in about less than 10% of sleep related breathing disorders. Remember that a combination or mixed, apnea also exists. The trouble with breathing due to difficulty with initiation of the respiratory cycle will be discussed first, but after we all understand what a respiratory cycle is.

Every breathing or respiratory cycle consists of two phases: an inspiratory phase (called inspiration) and an expiratory phase (called exhalation or expiration). Since expiration also refers to other things, some not so pleasant (e.g. death) I prefer to use the term exhalation rather than expiration. When listening to a patient's lung, I prefer to ask the patient to exhale rather than to expire. I would not want to shock the patient while he is being examined. During inspiration, room air is taken into the lungs. The amount of air inspired is known as a tidal volume. A normal breath consists of approximately 500 mL of air. 1000 mL is one liter, the size of many soft drink containers. In rough terms, to give you some perspective, one liter is approximately equal to 1 quart. Therefore, 500 mL is roughly equivalent to ½ of a quart. If you listen with a stethoscope you can actually hear air entering and leaving the chest cavity. An interesting consideration is that the time spent in inspiration is not equivalent to the time spent in exhalation. The exhalation phase actually lasts longer than inspiration. Again, in rough figures, if a normal respiratory cycle takes a total of 3 seconds to complete, 1 second would represent inhalation and 2 seconds would be exhalation. If you have emphysema or bronchitis, the amount spent in the exhalation phase is even longer. Room air consists of 21% oxygen. During inspiration the chest cavity enlarges as air is taken into the chest cavity. In this manner, a body receives its necessary oxygen supply. At the completion of the inspiratory portion of the cycle, there is actually a much larger volume of air present in the chest as compared to the beginning of the cycle. As noted above, this is approximately 500 mL. The main muscle of inspiration is the diaphragm which contracts and moves down towards the abdomen with inspiration, thus enlarging the chest cavity. Other important muscles include some of the muscles between the ribs, called intercostal muscles, and the muscles of the neck that also help expand the chest cavity by raising the ribs. This muscular action, as well as the time spent in each phase of the respiratory cycle, is normally not noted by the healthy person for, as the song says, breathing should be effortless, "like breathing out and breathing in." At the end of inspiration, the expiratory portion of the cycle begins. The muscles that were responsible for the expansion of the chest cavity relax. There are no muscles normally required for exhalation. Exhalation occurs primarily because of elasticity. The chest wall and surrounding structures, as well as the lungs, are elastic structures that have been stretched with inspiration and consequently have a tendency to recoil. Because of this, exhalation is normally simply a relaxation of the inspiratory muscles and other structures. The natural force of elasticity causes recoil of the chest wall and of the lungs expelling air from the lungs returning the chest structures to their normal resting state, albeit briefly. In other words, inhalation is normally active while exhalation is normally a passive process. You will soon discover how this normally well-coordinated effort is significantly disrupted in sleep related breathing disorders. By the way, we have already noted that inspiration provides the body with oxygen. What does exhalation do? Exhalation actually gets rid of carbon dioxide. The main function of the lungs is to provide gas exchange. Oxygen is taken in and carbon dioxide is expelled. The lungs have many functions, but gas exchange is the most important. Carbon dioxide is an end product of metabolism. Metabolism can be considered to be the sum total of the chemical reactions within the cells of the body that produce energy. The two end products when the body completely utilizes sugar for energy are carbon dioxide and water. In simplistic terms, the urinary system gets rid of water and the lungs get rid of carbon dioxide. If carbon dioxide accumulates in the body this would produce acid, as excess carbon dioxide is converted to acid if it remains in the body. Just as an aside, we noted that room air contains 21% oxygen. What makes up the rest of the components of room air? Actually, the vast majority is made up of nitrogen, normally an inert gas in the body. Nitrogen makes up 78% of room air. The remaining gases in room air consist of trace amounts of carbon dioxide, argon and other inert gases, as well as water. Now that we better understand the respiratory cycle and its function, we are almost prepared to look at problems with initiation of this important cycle.

Before proceeding further, however, I want to explain the expiratory phase of the respiratory cycle in a bit more detail for clarification. As we note above, the expiratory phase of the respiratory cycle is normally completely passive because of the elastic recoil of both the lungs and chest wall. This is true during quiet breathing such as at rest or during normal sleep. However during activities such as exercise, exhalation becomes an active process similar to inhalation. This process of exhalation then requires muscular effort. The muscles most important during active exhalation are the muscles of the abdomen. These are the muscles that make up the abdominal wall. When one coughs, defecates, or vomits these same muscles become important. Contraction of these muscles increases pressure in the abdomen causing the diaphragm to be pushed up towards the chest. Other muscles, such as some chest muscles, also come into play with forceful exhalation. However the most important muscles of active expiration are the abdominal muscles. We will come to see the importance of these abdominal muscles as we further analyze this fascinating topic of sleep apnea.

When lack of initiation of the respiratory cycle is the problem, the disease is referred to as central sleep apnea. These patients have difficulty with initiation of a breath when they are asleep. They tend to hold their breath periodically for some length of time. The problem is called "central" because it resides in the brain, actually the lower brain. The lower brain is the center for initiation of breathing. It is also part of the central nervous system. The brain is thus the pacemaker for our respiration and sets the respiratory rate and pattern. The concept of a pacemaker in the brain is akin to the concept of a pacemaker in the heart. The heart also has a pacemaker which regulates the heart rhythm and rate. The heart pacemaker function is better known to the general population than the brain pacemaker function. As the brain pacemaker is in the lower brain, this activity is normally carried out on a subconscious level. This means that it is not a voluntary or conscious act. If this respiratory drive is poorly transmitted from the lower brain to the muscles because of a neuromuscular illness, the breathing efforts may be diminished or even absent. If there is a problem with the brain, such as a tumor in the area of the pacemaker, then the initiation of a normal deep breath may be feeble or not occur at all. This is almost like a skipped heartbeat. A stroke in the same area of the brain can have a similar effect. Sometimes, there is an unstable pacemaker for breathing and this can also result in central sleep apnea. Sometimes medications may diminish the brain pacemaker function. Alcohol, narcotics, and sedatives can all be culprits under the right circumstances.

Central sleep apnea has a very interesting history. This is in part because it relates to literature. Central sleep apnea has been referred to in the medical literature as "Ondine's curse." European mythology and literature, primarily a combination of Greek mythology and German literature, have numerous references to Ondine, also known as Undine. Ondine is said to be a water nymph, whatever that is. She was extremely beautiful. According to mythology, all nymphs, beautiful or not, live forever unless they fall in love with a human and subsequently have an offspring. According to my version, beautiful Ondine fell in love with a medieval knight who promised her his undying love. For this Ondine gave up her immortality and became an ordinary human being like the rest of us. Sir Knight, however, failed to keep his promises. Because of Sir Knight's unfaithfulness, Ondine placed a curse on him telling him that as long as he was awake he would continue to breathe. However, when he would fall asleep his breathing would stop. He had to be conscious to control his breathing. Remember, Ondine gave up her immortality and some of her beauty for this guy. This conscious control of breathing became to be known as Ondine's curse. As we mentioned previously, breathing is normally a subconscious rather than a conscious endeavor. Transferring the breathing cycle from the subconscious to the conscious level is truly a curse. Ondine sure knew what she was doing. Poor Sir Knight must have been miserable! Basically, Ondine's curse refers to only central sleep apnea. At times it has been applied to sleep apnea in general.

The second type of sleep apnea is known as obstructive sleep apnea. This is an entirely different process from central sleep apnea. In this type of sleep apnea there is a very strong signal coming from the brain instructing the body to take a breath. There is nothing wrong with the pacemaker in the brain. The body, primarily the respiratory muscles, gets a very strong signal and attempts to vigorously comply. Consequently, there is a very strong attempt by the body to take a deep breath and complete the respiratory cycle. Exhalation thus becomes an active process in a person with obstructive sleep apnea. You will recall that in central sleep apnea there is either no signal, or a greatly diminished signal, given by the brain telling the body when to breathe. However, what happens in obstructive sleep apnea is that in spite of a very strong signal as well as a strong effort to breathe, patients are unable to breathe because the airway becomes obstructed. This is now a mechanical problem rather than a pacemaker problem. The patients' airways become obstructed in large part because of the relaxation of the upper airway muscles during sleep. This allows the soft tissues around the airway to relax; structures such as the tongue and soft palate consequently fall back closing down the airway. Obstructive sleep apnea actually does occur more in patients when they are lying on their backs. Often these patients try to avoid this position. When one is lying on his back, the forces of gravity have the greatest effect on collapsing the upper airway thereby causing obstruction. If these patients also have other structural problems, then the breathing problem can become even worse. Examples are greatly enlarged tonsils and adenoids, a retracted jawbone, or a smaller than normal diameter of the airway. These patients are instructed by their brain pacemaker to breathe and they actually want to breathe. Muscles of inspiration as well as muscles of expiration do not relax normally in obstructive sleep apnea. In fact they contract with great force. They are obeying the instructions of their pacemaker. Unfortunately, their efforts at breathing are overcome by mechanical resistance caused by loose, relaxed tissue surrounding the airway. The muscles and structures of the airway are loose and floppy and getting in the way of any air movement. Air movement is being obstructed. At times the patient will make such a severe effort at breathing, attempting to overcome the obstruction, that the motion of the chest and abdomen is quite evident to an observer. In fact, there is often lack of synchrony between the diaphragm, abdominal muscles, and the chest muscles. Normally the chest muscles, the diaphragm, and the abdominal muscles work synchronously to expand the chest cavity. In obstructive sleep apnea there may be what is known as paradoxical breathing where the diaphragm, the abdominal and the chest wall muscles are working against each other instead of with each other. In addition, because of the decreased opening of the airway and loose floppy tissue, there is significant noise associated with this type of breathing. The patient exhibits signs of snoring, choking, snorting and gasping. Interspersed, there may be periods of silence. This pattern of breathing is more common in patients that are heavier. However, slimmer people can also have obstructive sleep apnea. The correlation with heavier people also has a correlation with the literature. This time, however, instead of it being German literature it is the English literature that comes into play. I am referring to the Pickwick Papers by Charles Dickens. In this novel is found a character, fat boy Joe. Sleep physicians have long thought that fat boy Joe represented a patient with obstructive sleep apnea. Dickens described Joe as "fat and red faced boy in a state of somnolency." Somnolency, of course, means sleepy. Fat boy Joe repeatedly exhibited day time periods of sleepiness, or somnolency. Fat boy Joe appeared to be sleeping most of the day. This was obvious to all who knew fat boy Joe, especially Dickens. Early researchers studying obstructive sleep apnea consequently felt that Joe was the poster boy for obstructive sleep apnea. Hence, the German literature gives us the description for central sleep apnea while the English literature gives us the description for obstructive sleep apnea. Nice distinction; this helps us greatly in differentiating the two types of sleep apnea.

Regardless of the type of apnea, patients with sleep apnea tend to have excessive daytime somnolence, just like Joe. They do not feel refreshed from sleep. They tend to fall asleep during the day quite easily especially when there are minimal stimuli. Patients with sleep apnea might fall asleep at a red light, or, if the disease is bad enough, even while someone is talking to them. Those with obstructive sleep apnea may have prominent snoring and there is significant resistance to airflow. Patients will have a restless sleep, multiple awakenings during the night, and probably a morning headache. They will not feel refreshed when they wake up in the morning. Over time, there will probably be memory impairment and difficulty with concentration. The heart will also be affected. Abnormalities of the airways, as noted above, are more common in obstructive sleep apnea patients. This would include such anatomical problems as large tonsils and adenoids, a thick neck and obesity. Excess tissue and enlarged tonsils and adenoids significantly decrease the diameter of the airways. This predisposes to sleep apnea. Excess tissue is mostly due to excess fat, although sometimes it may be due to boggy, edematous tissue. In other words, excess fluid. Patients with a poorly pumping heart often experience increasing shortness of breath while lying down. If they stand up, the shortness of breath may improve. The medical explanation for this is that there is fluid buildup when people lie down, especially if they have large swollen edematous legs when standing. When these people lie down, the leg position moves from vertical to horizontal and the swelling of the legs normally diminishes significantly. This is because of hydrostatic pressure changes. Where does that excess water that was present in the legs go? The answer is that excess water goes from the legs into the vascular system and subsequently into the lungs and tissues of the body. In other words, fluid is redistributed throughout the body. Pumping the extra fluid places somewhat of an increased burden on the heart, especially noted when the heart is weak and having difficulty pumping blood. That is why someone with a weak heart may have less shortness of breath in the upright position then when lying down. In the upright position the blood pools in the lower extremities and there is less blood in the vascular system for the heart to pump and also less blood accumulates in the lungs and other tissues. This type of heart problem is sometimes called pump failure, or heart failure. An additional factor to consider is that when we assume the horizontal position, the abdominal contents plop down and push the diaphragm up into the chest. This may make it difficult for the person in this position to adequately take a deep breath. This is especially true in the sick or very obese individual. The chest cavity gets compressed, or squeezed, by the abdominal contents. People with sleep apnea also tend to have poorly controlled high blood pressure. The elevated blood pressure under these circumstances tends to respond poorly to blood pressure medication. There may be concern with driving as these patients have problems with concentration and also possibly falling asleep while driving. Acid reflux is also quite common. As you can tell, many medical problems can be correlated with sleep apnea. Multiple other body systems besides the lungs and upper airway may be involved. These may include the heart and vascular system, the brain and also the gastrointestinal tract.

Diagnosis of sleep apnea normally requires a sleep study. This is usually done in a sleep laboratory, although lately home sleep studies are becoming somewhat more popular. During the sleep study multiple measurements are taken of various bodily functions. These are referred to as leads. For instance, EEG leads (brain waves) are utilized to help determine levels or stages of sleep. The heart rate and type of rhythm is also monitored. Pulse oximetry (a measurement of oxygen content) is another important measurement since periods of significantly decreased oxygenation occur because of the multiple periods of apnea. Rib cage and abdominal efforts are also monitored. We mentioned above the importance of the chest wall and abdominal muscles in the respiratory cycle. Airflow is another aspect that is monitored. As many aspects, or leads, are included in this monitoring, the technique is referred to as polysomnography. "Poly" means many and the term basically means many recordings during sleep. When central apnea is present, these studies show that apnea consists of no air movement but also no effort at breathing. Chest rib motion and abdominal motion are absent during periods of apnea. In contrast, obstructive sleep apnea shows that during periods of apnea, there is no air movement even though there is significant effort at attempting to breathe. The chest muscles and abdominal muscles are working very hard in futile attempts to breathe. The diaphragm, the most important muscle of respiration, is also working. This great effort at breathing, as you now know, meets obstruction and consequently there is no air flow during periods of apnea. With both types of apnea, oxygenation suffers greatly. The following cartoons represent a simplified and idealized polysomnography. These are cartoons that I made up and do not represent an actual polysomnography. These squiggles are also not drawn to scale. The following cartoons show only essential portions of a polysomnography to better understand the basis of polysomnography. I have chosen only three leads to be shown, primarily air movement, rib cage or chest wall movement, and abdominal muscle movement leads. Besides the pulse oximetry lead, which is not depicted, these three leads are the most representative leads for understanding what is taking place in a sleep study. Many other leads that are normally utilized in polysomnography have been left out of my cartoons. That does not mean that the other leads are not important. These other leads were left out for simplicity's sake. Some of these important leads that have been left out include pulse oximetry tracing, EEG, and eye movements. Adding all these and other tracings would only confuse the issue.

We first present the cartoon which is a depiction of central sleep apnea.

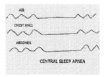

In this cartoon the top squiggle represents air movement. The second represents movement of the chest wall or rib cage. The third represents movement of abdominal muscles. All three are labeled. What we see here is that the patient first takes three breaths in and out. This is represented by the tracing showing the equivalent of three humps. Each hump represents one respiratory cycle, which is inspiration and exhalation. The air movement, the chest wall movement, and the abdominal movement are all similar. We subsequently see no evidence of movement for a period of time, and then movement resumes again in all three leads. The three basically flat lines in-between humps represents absence of air movement, absence of chest wall movement, and absence of abdominal movement. Consequently, this is a tracing of central sleep apnea. There is absence of breathing and the body is making no effort at taking a breath for a long period of time. Many breaths are skipped when apnea occurs. The apnea may last for 10 seconds or longer. Apnea is very evident and all leads show similar behavior. If we had shown a recording of the oxygen saturation (pulse oximeter), the tracing would be similar and there would be a significant drop in the oxygen saturation related to the prolonged period of apnea. This cartoon is typical of central sleep apnea and illustrates the essential diagnostic finding present in a typical polysomnography. We will now contrast these findings with a cartoon of the typical obstructive sleep apnea as seen in the next figure.

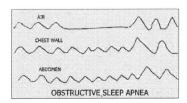

This cartoon is significantly different than the prior one. The same three leads are present, primarily air movement, chest wall or rib cage movement, and abdominal muscle movement. However, only the tracing representing the air movement is similar to the prior cartoon. We see that air movement squiggle shows a long straight line with humps at both ends. Again each hump represents a respiratory cycle, inspiration and exhalation. The long flat line again represents absence of air flow and consequently absence of breathing. In other words, apnea is present and is represented by the portion of the tracing that is flat. No air is getting in or out of the chest. The chest wall lead and the abdominal lead show strong contrast to the corresponding leads in the prior cartoon. We see that the humps continue throughout the tracing. There is no evidence of any flat line. This means that the muscles are attempting to breathe. However, in spite of these efforts, there is no evidence of air movement and consequently no evidence of breathing. The muscles are receiving the signal to breathe from the pacemaker in the lower brain. They want to breathe and this second cartoon tracing shows that the efforts continue but there is absence of air flow. The efforts are futile. No breathing or air exchange is taking place. If the above cartoon had included a lead for the pulse oximetry, we would see that decreased oxygen saturation would develop related to the period of apnea. This means that the amount of oxygen in the body is decreasing. Oxygen is being utilized but not being replaced. It would be a similar tracing for the cartoon showing central sleep apnea.

To sum up these homemade cartoons, it is important to note that both central sleep apnea and obstructive sleep apnea tracings show evidence of apnea, meaning primarily lack of breathing or lack of air movement. In central sleep apnea, when apnea takes place there is no movement in either the abdominal muscles or the chest wall muscles. There is also no movement of the diaphragm. All is quiet. In sharp contrast, during the period of apnea in obstructive sleep apnea there is significant movement of both the abdominal and chest wall muscles. The diaphragm is also working hard. As a matter of fact the movements may not be coordinated and the various muscles of respiration may work against each other. This is known as paradoxical breathing. All is not quiet in obstructive sleep apnea. Only the air movement is quiet. Some people look at these two types of apnea as, "won't breathe" as opposed to "can't breathe." Of course people with central sleep apnea "won't breathe." People with obstructive sleep apnea "can't breathe." This is another easy way to differentiate the two types.

As can be deduced from the above discussion, the diagnosis of sleep apnea normally requires polysomnography. This is known as a sleep study. The physician interpreting the polysomnography will be looking for periods of apnea and quantitating the episodes of apnea to estimate the severity of the disease. Just to complicate matters slightly, the interpreting physician would be looking not only for periods of apnea, but also for episodes of what are known as hypopnea. You now know that apnea refers to the complete cessation of air movement. Hypopnea represents a new term for you. Hypopnea is somewhat more difficult to define. Hypopnea is very important, but its definition may vary slightly from physician to physician. Basically, hypopnea represents a diminished, but not complete, cessation of air flow. There is a definite loss in the quality of breathing, but breathing does not completely stop. Associated with this diminished air flow is also evidence of loss of oxygen saturation. Additionally, both hypopnea and apnea are normally terminated by some decrease in the stage of sleep. This implies that there is evidence of arousal of the patient at the conclusion of both an apnea episode and a hypopnea episode. This evidence of arousal can be found in the EEG leads of the sleep study. The big advantage of polysomnography is that the activities being recorded by all the various leads, all at the same time, can be correlated. Both apnea and hypopnea contribute to interruption of sleep. Similarly, both are coordinated with loss of oxygen saturation. Consequently, both of these types of sleep interruption are of significant importance. Only one shows complete cessation of air flow, but both show evidence of arousal and evidence of oxygen deprivation. These are the hallmarks of a fitful and non-restful sleep. Often and gradually, over a period possibly of years, these hallmarks take their toll on the human body.

The physician interpreting any sleep study has many objectives including quantitating the severity of any sleep related breathing disorder found. Consequently, he will attempt to quantify every disturbance related to quality of sleep. Included in this would be the sum total of all the episodes of apnea plus hypopnea. He will actually count every episode, every event. He will also determine the total length of sleep by analyzing the various leads. He will determine what is known as the apnea-hypopnea index. This index defines the total number of episodes of apnea plus hypopnea that occur per hour. This important index is abbreviated as AHI. Apnea and hypopnea events are thus treated as being essentially the same thing. The physician then has a simple number recording the total number of apnea plus hypopnea events occurring per hour of sleep, the AHI. That simple number can be used to grade the severity of the illness. It can also be used for comparison purposes between the study that is being interpreted and any other study that that patient may have had or will have. Remember, the physician can grade the severity of the sleep apnea by the number of episodes that occur. Can you believe that severe sleep apnea may show as many as 30 or more episodes per hour? Wow, that is an average of one episode every two minutes! How can anybody with this many episodes ever get enough sleep?

Let's take a closer look at arousal. Arousals are important components of the sleep cycle. We noted above that arousal from sleep may occur multiple times during sleep and, as a matter of fact, multiple times within minutes even. By arousal, we do not mean that the patient completely wakes up. What we mean is that the stage of sleep is not as deep as it would otherwise be. The patient goes from a deeper stage of sleep to a lighter stage. A definite downgrade in the quality of sleep occurs with each arousal. Arousals cause changes to occur. Arousal necessarily stimulates the nervous system. This is good, because the muscles that become relaxed during apnea now regain their normal function. Remember we noticed earlier that the muscles of the upper airway, primarily the tongue, soft palate and the muscles of the surrounding structures all relax during sleep. The airway relaxes and actually collapses during sleep. The collapsibility of the airway is an important factor in the production of obstruction in sleep apnea. Arousal helps reverse this relaxation. The muscles consequently tighten and the airway opens. The collapsibility disappears from the upper airway. The patient is now able to breathe and exchange air. The lungs have regained their ability to carry out their normal function. Although frequent arousals are not good for sleep quality, they are good for oxygenation. The deterioration in oxygenation improves because of the state of arousal. However, arousal, through its stimulation of the nervous system, causes an increase in substances, such as adrenaline, which may have their own adverse outcomes. Adrenaline, also known as epinephrine, can lead to both an elevated heart rate and an elevated blood pressure. There may even be irregular heartbeats. In arousal these factors may actually amount to a two edged sword. The beneficial side is an improvement in oxygenation. The detrimental side may be potential harmful effects on the heart as well as the interruption in the quality of sleep. Here again, over a long period of time, mainly years, the detrimental effects may take their toll on the body.

We will now look more deeply into what type of person we would expect to develop sleep apnea. The patient is usually a male, although postmenopausal females may also have similar problems. We are already aware that people who are obese (especially if they have a large neck) and those that have abnormalities of the upper airways are predisposed to the development of obstructive sleep apnea. As noted previously, obesity is not an absolute requirement and many that are not considered obese may still have sleep apnea. Tongue size may also be of importance. This may be suspected if there are ridge markings from teeth on the tongue. People can store fat even in the tongue. People who snore excessively are also predisposed. As a matter of fact, snoring is considered an essential component in the diagnosis of sleep apnea. Patients normally are not aware of snoring. In patients with sleep apnea, snoring may occur even prior to onset of sleep; snoring may occur during periods of drowsiness. During sleep, snoring may be interrupted by periods of silence, reflecting apnea in most cases. Although snoring is considered to be an essential component for the diagnosis, it is important to remember that many people snore but do not have sleep apnea. Moreover, such factors as alcohol and medication can also contribute to the production of snoring. Advancing age is also a risk factor. This may in part be because the disease is often a slowly progressive type of disease and consequently often noted as one ages. People with thyroid disease may have some predisposition to sleep apnea. People with neuromuscular difficulties may have a predisposition, especially to the central type of sleep apnea.

Now that we know what sleep apnea is and what type of people are predisposed to this ailment, we are ready to explore the presentation of someone that has sleep apnea.

Basically, this means the signs and symptoms of sleep apnea. One of my prior books entitled *RECOGNIZING SYMPTOMS OF COMMON LUNG DISEASES* describes in detail the differences between signs and symptoms. Basically, symptoms express what the patient's problems are from the patient's perspective. These are consequently subjective findings. For instance, a headache is a subjective finding, therefore a symptom. There is no way a physician can know that a patient has a headache simply by examining the patient. In other words this is not an objective finding. An example of an objective finding would be a skipped heartbeat or an abnormal EKG. These are findings that are objective, meaning independent of patient interpretation. A subjective finding is a symptom while an objective finding is a sign. Both symptoms and signs are necessary in making a diagnosis, any diagnosis - not just sleep apnea.

You will recall from the *Introduction to Sleep Apnea* chapter, we began the discussion by noting a number of scenarios. These scenarios are actually what one may expect in real life if one has a significant problem with sleep apnea. These scenarios represent some of the signs and symptoms of people that have sleep apnea. We will now examine these more closely.

People with sleep apnea at times have what appears to be unexplained behavior. Sometimes, while sitting and waiting at a red light, they may doze off or actually fall asleep. Consequently when the light changes to green they may just sit there and the person behind them might get annoyed. This, of course, is because of excessive daytime somnolence. These patients fail to obtain a restful sleep during the night. There is no restorative function to their sleep. They are not refreshed in the morning. As we have noted they may have many periods of arousal throughout the night. Periods of arousal have both a beneficial and a detrimental effect, especially over the long term, on the body as was just recently explained. The short term effect however is primarily excessive daytime somnolence leading to activities such as described. As you now know fat boy Joe is the poster boy for this. Fortunately, fat boy Joe never drove a car. Excessive daytime somnolence and snoring are normally considered to be two common and essential components for the diagnosis of obstructive sleep apnea.

Morning headache, on the other hand, is much less common and not essential for the diagnosis. However, the rationale for a morning headache is quite interesting. You will recall from the cartoons that apnea is represented as a flat line, a time when no breathing takes place. You are aware that during this period of a flat line formation in the cartoon, the oxygen content of the blood is being depleted because there is no gas exchange. As a consequence of lack of breathing, one other component of gas exchange needs to be considered. I am referring to carbon dioxide which builds up during apnea periods. Carbon dioxide is not expelled during periods of apnea. Morning headache is attributed to the buildup of carbon dioxide during these periods. What happens is that carbon dioxide causes an increase in the size of the vessels in the brain, a process known as vasodilation. This contributes to increased pressure in the head and consequently to the headache.

People with obstructive sleep apnea often have complaints consistent with insomnia. However, they appear to fall asleep relatively quickly. The time one takes to fall asleep in medical terms is known as sleep latency. In fact, sleep latency is normally short in patients with sleep apnea. Thus, the complaint of insomnia given by patients with obstructive sleep apnea technically refers to the frequent periods of arousal and not to inability to fall asleep. There is a difference. As noted in the scenario where one is walking by his friend's home on a summer evening, during these periods patients often make unusual sounds such as choking, gasping and may also become restless. All these factors contribute to excessive daytime somnolence, contributing to factors already mentioned such as drowsiness while driving and possibly increase in car accidents. In fact, drowsiness can also contribute to difficulty with work performance, school performance and other similar factors. Sleep physicians often use a short questionnaire to assess possibility of dozing off under various conditions. This is known as the Epworth Sleepiness Scale. Questions asked refer to a probability of dozing off during various activities such as watching TV, sitting or talking to someone, or after lunch. This questionnaire is a helpful but not an absolute indication of the state of sleepiness.

Another prominent symptom of patients with sleep apnea is excessive urination during the night. Urination at night, in medical terms, is known as nocturia. Patients have to get up to urinate multiple times. Often patients have coexisting disease and therefore may not realize that the excessive urination may be caused by sleep apnea. As an example, as you know sleep apnea is correlated with advancing age; likewise for diabetes and prostate problems. Consequently, both of these other problems can also contribute to excessive urination during the night. The poor patient with obstructive sleep apnea may have multiple reasons for waking from sleep throughout the night. The lowering of the oxygen concentration because of sleep apnea and the increase in fluid because of the horizontal position are believed to be responsible for the excessive urination.

There is a correlation between sleep apnea and many other diseases such as high blood pressure. More recently even diabetes and cardioembolic stroke have been noted to correlate with sleep apnea. You may recall that one of our scenarios referred to difficult to control high blood pressure. Elevated and difficult to control blood pressure has long been known to be present in sleep apnea patients. The medical term for elevated blood pressure is hypertension. Often patients are treated aggressively for hypertension without any significant improvement. For example, a patient may be on as many as three different medications for the treatment of elevated blood pressure without any significant benefit. Improvement in these particular cases takes place only after treatment for obstructive sleep apnea is also undertaken. Irregular heartbeat, known as arrhythmia, has also correlated with sleep apnea. You may recall in the discussion about arousal that we mentioned that during arousal there is a release of substances such as epinephrine that may contribute to irregular heartbeats. A number of different abnormal heart rhythms have been attributed to obstructive sleep apnea, not the least of which is atrial fibrillation, an all too frequent rhythm disturbance. Atrial fibrillation has multiple causes. I am sure you have seen the various advertisements on television regarding atrial fibrillation and certain medications. Consequently, as previously mentioned, sleep apnea can have a significant effect on cardiac health.

Chapter 3: DISEASES WITH SIMILARITY TO SLEEP APNEA

In analyzing diseases, physicians frequently find many similarities between diseases. In order to arrive at one diagnosis, physicians have to consider both the similarities and the differences between specific diseases. In medical thinking, this process is known as differential diagnosis. To better understand an individual disease, how that disease is similar and how it is different from other related diseases sharpens one's knowledge. It also helps to better define the disease process. In spite of detailed medical knowledge, it is not always possible to identify a specific disease. At times the medical diagnoses made actually represent a group of diseases, rather than one specific disease. This conclusion may be evident when the term is something similar to "overlap syndrome" but not as obvious when that term is "idiopathic." As politicians do not appear to admit to, words do have meaning. We will now review some of these diseases related to sleep apnea.

Two important findings in sleep apnea are excessive daytime somnolence and snoring. Many diseases beside sleep apnea can present with these findings. Some of the diseases that may mimic sleep apnea include asthma and other lung problems, narcolepsy, restless leg syndrome, heart failure, as well as gastric reflux. Each of these diseases, discussed below, may contribute to poor sleep quality and consequently mimic sleep apnea. Some of the causes of poor sleep quality may be due to medications or various other reasons, and not necessarily to a disease state. An example of a condition that is not necessarily a disease is shift work, a common cause of sleepiness and poor sleep quality.

It is not unusual for patients with asthma and other lung diseases to awaken during the night. Often they wake up short of breath and wheezing. There are a number of reasons for this occurrence including fluctuations in the airway diameter and in the level of medications. Similarly, patients with emphysema and bronchitis will have variations in sleep status, including variations in the oxygen saturation. These symptoms are not necessarily specific to asthma and other lung conditions. We noted above that persons with congestive heart failure (pump failure) had redistribution of fluid from the legs to other organs such as the lungs. You will recall that the fluid shift was due to changes in position from the vertical to horizontal. Increased fluid under these conditions in the lungs causes shortness of breath and awakenings during the night. Under these conditions without further studies, it may be difficult to separate heart from lung problems. As a matter of fact, there is a condition that can be described as "cardiac asthma." This is where excessive fluid in the lungs causes wheezing in a person who does not have asthma. This fact has led to the medical statement that "all that wheezes is not asthma."

Narcolepsy is a rare but alarming disorder. It tends to occur in much younger patients. Narcolepsy, like other diseases mentioned, is associated with significant sleepiness; but it also has other, sometimes alarming problems, including sleep associated paralysis and hallucinations. Narcolepsy has a tendency to run in families. The problem with narcolepsy concerns REM sleep and consequent loss of the normal ordinary sleep rhythm. Manifestations of REM sleep can occur inappropriately during periods of wakefulness. During these periods, which can occur suddenly, the patient loses muscle tone and can even fall from a standing position. These are known as "drop attacks." Other times, the manifestation may be more subtle such as a muscle twitch. These episodes are known as cataplexy and can be precipitated by emotions, such as anger or even laughing. There is no loss of consciousness. Not all patients with narcolepsy have these episodes. The predominant problem is excessive sleepiness. Hallucinations consist of vivid dreams during REM activity, which as noted, can occur even when the patient is fully awake. These patients can wake up from sleep with sleep paralysis. At that time they are unable to move, and actually have paralysis. This also relates to REM associated sleep. For all these multiple reasons, narcolepsy can be an alarming disorder.

Restless leg syndrome also leads to excessive sleepiness. These patients have abnormal sensations. They complain of having a feeling of creeping or crawling in their legs. This feeling occurs typically near the hour of sleep. Inactivity can make these feelings worse, and patients with restless leg syndrome often increase activity to attempt to relieve this annoying feeling. They developed an urge to move their legs. Because these episodes often occur at time of sleep, they contribute to the disordered sleep. Restless leg syndrome is more prominent in pregnancy, people on dialysis, and people with iron deficiency. There is also a familial correlation. You may have seen some of the TV advertisements for medications used in the treatment of restless legs syndrome. These days, just about anything is advertised on television, including medications people want you to request from your doctor.

The last disease mentioned above that can mimic sleep apnea is gastric reflux. The reflux of acid from the stomach can disrupt sleep and lead to excessive daytime sleepiness. This is a common problem, but differentiation from sleep apnea is normally not difficult.

Chapter 4: FACTS YOU SHOULD KNOW ABOUT THE MEDICAL TREATMENT OF SLEEP APNEA

There are a number of approaches that can be taken in treating the problem of sleep apnea. Your personal physician may choose one or more of these, depending on the circumstances. Remember, a primary goal of treatment is the prevention of the many long-term adverse events that can occur as a result of sleep apnea. There are long and short-term complications that need to be considered during treatment. These adverse events could include loss of memory, personality changes, difficulties with work or school, or cardiac damage. The latter requires adequate control of blood pressure and weight. As noted previously, controlling blood pressure might involve not only adequate blood pressure medication but also adequate control of sleep apnea. Adequate control of weight may even call for bariatric surgery. Occasionally, controlling diabetes may also be a factor to correlate with obstructive sleep apnea. Obstructive sleep apnea has been implicated to cause increased insulin resistance. Treatment of atrial fibrillation may need assessment and treatment of sleep apnea. Therefore adequate treatment of sleep apnea implies more than simply treatment of sleep apnea itself.

The most popular treatment for sleep apnea involves either CPAP or BIPAP. This is usually the standard approach of pulmonologists and is known as positive airway pressure. Basically, this method of treatment involves breathing against resistance. Resistance is placed in the airway from the outside through the mouth or nose in order to keep the airway open and free of obstruction. Positive pressure acts as a "splint" for the airway. This helps keep the airway open both during inhalation and exhalation. This resistance is known as positive airway pressure and requires some sort of mask. The term positive airway pressure is used to designate that the breathing cycle has positive pressure from beginning to end of the cycle. Normally inhalation is negative during the breathing cycle. It may be helpful to review the section on the breathing cycle presented in a prior chapter. Inhalation normally occurs because the chest cavity moves out and the diaphragm drops down into the abdomen and enlarges the chest cavity. This produces a negative pressure within the chest, basically sucking air into the chest cavity. That is why I stated that normally inhalation is negative during the breathing cycle. With positive pressure the air is basically pushed into the chest during inspiration. Contrast this with negative pressure breathing. An example of negative pressure breathing is the old iron lung. You may have seen pictures of polio wards in the 1950s. These wards had large tanks each of which covered practically the whole body of the patient, except for the head and neck. The tanks would provide negative pressure, expanding the chest cavity and letting air flow into the chest. Because of the availability of positive pressure ventilation, these tanks are no longer used.

CPAP is an acronym for continuous positive airway pressure. This was just explained. Remember, with positive pressure breathing the airway is kept positive both during inhalation and exhalation. The other term used in treatment of sleep apnea is BiPAP. BiPAP is slightly different. It implies two levels of pressure or, as some people say, bi-level pressure. What happens with BiPAP is that there is a different pressure for inspiration as opposed to exhalation. Both pressures remain positive. Pressure for inhalation is set at a higher level than for exhalation. Either CPAP or BiPAP may be used in treatment of sleep apnea, with CPAP being the more commonly used. Thus, CPAP delivers a constant amount of pressure or resistance to the airway. This pressure remains constant throughout both inhalation and exhalation. How much resistance the patients have to breathe against is normally measured in what is called a titration study. During this study increasing resistance is utilized while a patient is having a sleep study. When the sleep study shows that there is the least evidence of apnea at a certain pressure, that level of resistance, or pressure, is chosen and continued on an outpatient basis. The patients normally wear a facial or nasal mask that allows the continuation of the same level of pressure during sleep at home. Some current machines are more sophisticated and can have some role in adjusting the pressures without human input. This positive airway pressure has been shown to be effective in both central and obstructive sleep apnea. BiPAP may be necessary when that level of pressure is too high and consequently difficult for the patient to comfortably utilize. At that time, a higher inspiratory pressure and a lower pressure with exhalation can be better tolerated. This way the patient will have less, but adequate resistance with exhalation. BiPAP may also be better suited for the patient that has central sleep apnea. If the patient does not initiate a breath, a BiPAP machine will push air in and perform a modified breathing cycle. The BiPAP can even be set at a certain backup rate to help maintain air exchange. For instance it can be set at a rate of 10, basically assuring a minimum of 10 breaths per minute. BiPAP consequently becomes a form of ventilatory control or support.

Another method of treatment involves oral appliances. This is usually the treatment applied by dentists. There are a number of these appliances and they aim to hold the tongue in place and/or also to help keep the jaw in place and not fall back towards the throat. The idea is to stabilize the lower jaw and tongue in a forward position, helping to maintain an open airway. Similar to CPAP or BiPAP, these appliances seek to keep an open airway during sleep. These types of appliances have also been shown to be of benefit, especially in patients with less severe sleep apnea. These appliances may also be of benefit when someone is unable to tolerate a CPAP or BiPAP mask.

Surgical treatment has been another approach to treatment of obstructive sleep apnea. This, of course, is much more complicated than either of the above two choices. It is usually not the procedure of first choice, and results may vary. Surgical treatment can involve procedures such as a tracheotomy or a resection of the various soft tissues of the mouth and throat. Significantly enlarged tonsils and adenoids may rarely make surgical treatment an early or first choice. This is rare in adults.

A number of medications have also been used. Success however has been less than optimal. Some of the medications that have been tried are acetazolamide, theophylline, doxapram, and protriptyline. None of these, or numerous other medications, have as yet been able to replace the above three approaches. Sometimes medication can be used in conjunction with the other approaches.

A rather unusual treatment has been attempted by some and at least deserves mention at this point. Some people have suggested that with very mild obstructive sleep apnea so-called positional therapy may be of benefit. They suggest that positioning of pillows or placement of an object on the back during the night, such as a tennis ball sewn into a pajama top, may be helpful. I guess it would not hurt to try.

Sometimes central sleep apnea needs further treatment. A ventilator is occasionally necessary when the disease is severe enough. Ventilators are further discussed in the chapter concerning *RESPIRATORY FAILURE* in my book *WHAT YOU SHOULD KNOW ABOUT ASTHMA AND OTHER LUNG DISEASE*. Another one of my books called, *THE VENTILATOR*

DEPENDENT PATIENT: END OF LIFE ISSUE? also discusses ventilators and ventilator patients. Another technique that is sometimes considered in treating central sleep apnea patients is nerve stimulation, such as stimulation of the phrenic nerve. The phrenic nerve is a long nerve that goes from the brain to the diaphragm. The phrenic nerve instructs the diaphragm to breathe, normally carrying the message from the brain. This procedure is, of course, a highly skilled surgical procedure and is not always readily available.

An interesting old treatment seldom used today is the rocking bed. Sleep apnea patients are placed on a bed that rocks during the night. The rocking is not side to side but from head to toe. What happens is, as the patients are raised to greater than 40 degrees, the diaphragm drops down and the patients consequently take in a breath. When the patients are moved back to slightly below the horizontal position, the diaphragm moves back up and air is expelled. This is an interesting technique that may work for central sleep apnea but it is very rarely, if ever, used today.

Returning to the medical treatment of obstructive sleep apnea, emphasis should again be made of the need for weight loss in obese patients. With weight loss there should be improvement in the episodes of apnea.

Chapter 5: WHAT DOES ALL THIS MEAN FOR YOU?

If you have evidence of significant snoring or if you have been told that you appear to hold your breath while sleeping, sleep apnea is a consideration. This is especially true if you are sleepy throughout the day, if you easily fall asleep such as while you are sitting at a red light, if you do not feel refreshed in the morning, or if you are having difficulty with memory or concentration. If some or all of these things appear to be present, sleep apnea is a strong consideration. According to medical literature, sleep apnea diagnosis is often not made, or greatly delayed. To avoid this, sleep apnea should be kept in mind when the above symptoms are noticed. If you drink alcohol, especially before going to sleep, your symptoms might worsen. Alcohol may induce sleep, but it is followed by a very strong and prolonged arousal period contributing to a sleepless night. Additionally, alcohol contributes to loss of muscle tone of the upper airway during sleep. This contributes further to obstruction during sleep. If you are obese, weight loss should be a priority. If you have problems with tonsils and adenoids, you should have this evaluated by your physician.

If a diagnosis of sleep apnea is made, you should make every attempt to comply with your physician's advice and utilize the known methods of treatment, most likely starting with positive airway pressure. Remember, treatment is often a lifelong undertaking. You should make every effort to use your mask every night while asleep. This is true even during vacations. You are attempting to avoid short-term problems as well as long-term complications. A large variety of masks are available. If one is uncomfortable, there are many others you can choose. It is important that you get just the right fit and comfort. Additionally, before using the mask throughout the first night, a brief trial for about 30 minutes during the day might help you ease into continuous use of the mask. If you lose a significant amount of weight you may need further sleep studies, either to see if sleep apnea is still present or if you now need different pressures. You should be aware of the actual pressures that are best for you, and if you end up in a hospital you should be able to tell them what pressure you use in your mask at home. You would be surprised at the number of patients that I have seen who use CPAP or BiPAP at home on a regular basis, and yet have no idea of the pressures they have been using. A way around this may be that there are some CPAP machines that are self-adjusting, so called "smart" CPAP devices. Patients often complain of drying and lack of humidity in the airway when using CPAP or BiPAP. Under these conditions, humidity may be necessary and is normally relatively easy to incorporate into the system.

If you have sleep apnea and surgery is being contemplated, surgery for any reason and not just for sleep apnea, there are certain important considerations that you should be aware of. You will recall that part of the risk factors for sleep apnea was the basic structure of the neck and upper airway. People with thick necks and crowded upper airways are predisposed to sleep apnea. These are the exact same people that may be predisposed to complications during intubation or extubation when these procedures are necessary for the surgery or other medical reason. To clarify, intubation is the placement of a tube into the upper airway. This is often necessary for surgery so that the anesthesiologist can provide adequate oxygenation and ventilation throughout the surgical procedure. Sleep apnea patients with upper airway abnormalities present an increased challenge to the anesthesiologist, especially when the tube is being introduced (intubation) and when it is being removed (known as extubation). An inadequate airway is a dangerous situation. Because of sedation and potential swelling, the interval after removal of the tube can be crucial. The anesthesiologist and nursing staff will keep a close watch on your breathing while you are in the Recovery Room. By the way, what is wrong with the designation of Recovery Room? These rooms are now called PACCU, or post anesthesia critical care unit. The same holds for the old designation of ER, now changed to ED to designate a department, not simply a room. A room wasn't good enough for these guys. ED now sounds like part of the ads normally seen on television for certain kinds of pills. By the way, ED has also been associated with sleep apnea. Since I am not a urologist, I do not feel competent to discuss that topic. Watch your television for additional information.

Chapter 6: SUMMARY

Sleep is not a quiet state where nothing is going on. Sleep is composed of many events, most of which are not visible to the naked eye. A respiratory cycle consists of inhalation and exhalation. Ordinarily, inhalation produces a negative pressure, helping suck air into the chest cavity. Exhalation expels air from the chest cavity and at rest is attributed to elastic recoil of the chest structures. The main function of the lungs is exchange of air, taking in oxygen and giving off carbon dioxide. Orderly sleep is cyclical in nature. Sleep is composed of states, primarily REM sleep and non-REM sleep. In addition sleep is composed of stages of sleep, light sleep to deep sleep. Dreams and other activities occur during REM sleep. Arousal can refer to either complete awakening or moving from a deeper stage of sleep to a lesser. Episodes of apnea and hypopnea are very important events during a sleep study. These events can occur as often as 30 times per hour when severe sleep apnea is present.

Sleep apnea is a complex disease. Two main forms exist, central sleep apnea and obstructive sleep apnea. Obstructive sleep apnea is by far the more common type of apnea that people have. Occasionally patients can have both, but the obstructive significantly predominates. Another way to look at the two types is "can't breathe" and "won't breathe." Also remember Ondine's curse and fat boy Joe. Excessive daytime sleepiness and snoring are hallmarks of sleep apnea. Long-term complications of sleep apnea include confusion, disorientation, difficulties at work or in school, and cardiovascular events.

Treatment is directed towards prevention of long-term damage and avoidance of daytime sleepiness. Positive pressure is able to treat most cases of sleep apnea. If central sleep apnea is extremely severe, mechanical ventilation may be needed. I prefer the rocking bed, although this is essentially no longer in fashion. Weight loss is important. If you are unable to concentrate or if you fall asleep readily, consideration should be given to not driving a car or doing other tasks that require concentration. You may have to give up these activities until your treatment has become effective.

Questions

1. The most appropriate description of a Tidal Volume is that
   a. it is the total amount of air in the chest
   b. it is the pressure on a CPAP machine
   c. it is normally about 500 mL

2. Name three types of treatment for sleep apnea.
   a. _____
   b. _____
   c. _____

3. The type of apnea associated with fat boy Joe is _____ sleep apnea.

4. True or False
   a. __ At rest both inhalation and exhalation are active processes.
   b. __ The main function of the lungs is gas exchange.
   c. __ Most of room air is composed of oxygen.
   d. __ The body has pacemakers in both the brain and the heart.
   e. __ Sir Knight (the recipient of Ondine's curse according to my version) had obstructive sleep apnea.
   f. __ Paradoxical breathing normally occurs in central sleep apnea.
   g. __ Narcolepsy is a disease of old age.

h. ___An enlarged tongue may be an indication of obstructive sleep apnea.
i. ___ If fat boy Joe were alive today, he would make a good truck driver.
j. ___ Symptoms are objective findings by a physician.
k. ___Cataplexy is found in obstructive sleep apnea.
l. ___Pulse oximetry provides some detail about the amount of oxygen in the body.
m. ___ Signs are more important than Symptoms.

5. Monitoring air flow is the same as monitoring _____ during a sleep study.

6. If a respiratory cycle lasts 3 seconds, inhalation would last_____ second(s) while exhalation would last_____ second(s).

7. The main muscle of inhalation is the _____.

8. For a person with Ondine's curse to breathe, he must be _____.

9. _____ breathing is when the abdominal muscles, the diaphragm, and chest wall muscles are not working synchronously.

10. Apnea causes oxygen to _____ and carbon dioxide to _____.

11. Polysomnography refers to monitoring during a _____ study.

12. Apnea refers to _____ of air flow while Hypopnea refers to _____ air flow.

13. Adrenaline (epinephrine) causes an _____ in heart rate and an _____ in blood pressure.

14. "Cardiac asthma" refers to _____ fluid in the lungs causing _____ similar to asthma.

15. People with restless leg syndrome may have _____ deficiency anemia.

16. Atrial fibrillation is an _____ heart rhythm.

17. CPAP is an acronym for _____ _____ _____ _____.

18. A rocking bed may possibly have some use in the treatment of _____ sleep apnea.

19. BiPAP has a higher pressure for _____ than for _____.

Answers and Discussion

1. The most appropriate description of a Tidal Volume is that
    a. it is the total amount of air in the chest
    b. it is the pressure on a CPAP machine
    c. it is normally about 500 mL - this is the correct answer - the Tidal Volume is the amount of air that is taken in during a normal resting breath.

2. Name three types of treatment for sleep apnea.
    a. _____ positive pressure - CPAP and/or BiPAP
    b. _____ oral appliances
    c. _____ surgery

3. The type of apnea associated with fat boy Joe is **obstructive** sleep apnea.

4. True or False
    a. __ At rest both inhalation and exhalation are active processes. **False** – only inhalation is active; exhalation is passive and due to elastic recoil
    b. __ The main function of the lungs is gas exchange. **True** – the lungs have many functions but gas exchange is most important
    c. __ Most of room air is composed of oxygen. **False** – oxygen is the most important but not the most abundant

d. __ The body has pacemakers in both the brain and the heart. **True** – the brain is the pacemaker for respiration; the heart pacemaker controls heart rhythm

e. __ Sir Knight (the recipient of Ondine's curse according to my version) had obstructive sleep apnea. **False** – Ondine's curse is the conscious control of respiration and concerns central sleep apnea

f. __ Paradoxical breathing normally occurs in central sleep apnea. **False** – paradox occurs when respiratory muscles are not in sync

g. __ Narcolepsy is a disease of old age. **False** – narcolepsy occurs in young people

h. __An enlarged tongue may be an indication of obstructive sleep apnea. **True** – enlarged tongue can contribute to obstruction

i. __ If fat boy Joe were alive today, he would make a good truck driver. **False** – he would be too sleepy to drive and would cause accidents

j. __ Symptoms are objective findings by a physician. **False** – symptoms are subjective findings

k. __Cataplexy is found in obstructive sleep apnea. **False** – Cataplexy is the sudden loss of muscle tone. It may be found in narcolepsy and is triggered by emotion (e.g. laughing). It is not found in sleep apnea.

l. __Pulse oximetry provides some detail about the amount of oxygen in the body. **True** – pulse oximetry measures the oxygen saturation of hemoglobin

m. __ Signs are more important than Symptoms. **False** – both signs and symptoms are important – signs are objective and symptoms are subjective

5. Monitoring air flow is the same as monitoring **breathing** during a sleep study. – if there is no airflow, there is no breathing

6. If a respiratory cycle lasts 3 seconds, inhalation would last **one** second(s) while exhalation would last **two** second(s). – Exhalation lasts longer than inhalation

7. The main muscle of inhalation is the **diaphragm**. - The diaphragm expands the chest cavity during inhalation

8. For a person with Ondine's curse to breathe, he must be **awake**. – Remember, Ondine stated that he would quit breathing if he fell asleep

9. **Paradoxical** breathing is when the abdominal muscles, the diaphragm, and chest wall muscles are not working synchronously. - This occurs in obstructive sleep apnea

10. Apnea causes oxygen to **decrease** and carbon dioxide to **increase**. – Because no air exchange takes place during apnea

11. Polysomnography refers to monitoring during a **sleep** study. -Many leads are utilized during a sleep study

12. Apnea refers to **absence** of air flow while Hypopnea refers to **diminished** air flow. - Both cause decreased oxygen and some arousal

13. Adrenaline (epinephrine) causes an **increase** in heart rate and an **increase** in blood pressure. - adrenalin release stimulates the heart and blood pressure

14. "Cardiac asthma" refers to **increased** fluid in the lungs causing **wheezing** similar to asthma. - Remember, all that wheezes is not asthma

15. People with restless leg syndrome may have **iron** deficiency anemia. - It is a good idea to have your iron level checked if you have restless leg syndrome

16. Atrial fibrillation is an **abnormal** heart rhythm. - This abnormal heart rhythm is occasionally associated with sleep apnea

17. CPAP is an acronym for **Continuous Positive Airway Pressure.** - With normal breathing, part of the respiratory cycle has negative pressure - with CPAP the pressure is positive throughout

18. A rocking bed may possibly have some use in the treatment of **Central** sleep apnea. - Seldom, if ever, used today

19. BiPAP has a higher pressure for **inhalation** than for **exhalation**. - Has two different pressures - also called Bilevel

INDEX

active state of sleep, 17
adrenaline. *See* epinephrine
alcohol, 35, 51
apnea, 19
Apnea Hypopnea Index, 33
asthma, 42
atrial fibrillation, 39
BIPAP, 45
brain waves, 28
carbon dioxide, 22
cardiac asthma, 42
cataplexy, 42
central sleep apnea, 19, 23, 24, 48, 49, 55
Charles Dickens, 26
collapsibility of the airway, 34
CPAP, 45, 46, 47, 52, 57, 59, 61, 65
diaphragm, 21
differential diagnosis, 41
dreams, 17
elasticity, 21
epinephrine, 34, 39, 59, 64
excessive urination, 38
gas exchange, 21, 37, 57, 61
gastric reflux, 43
heart failure, 27
hypertension, 39
hypopnea, 32, 33, 55
interruption of sleep, 33
intubation, 52
iron lung, 46
large neck, 35
morning headache, 37
muscles of the abdomen, 22
muscles of the upper airway, 34
narcolepsy, 42
nitrogen, 22
non-REM sleep, 17
obstructive sleep apnea, 19, 24, 26, 29, 47, 48, 49, 55
Ondine, 23
Ondine's curse, 19, 24, 55, 57, 62
oral appliances, 47
paradoxical breathing, 25, 32
Pickwick Papers, 26
Pickwickian syndrome, 19
polysomnography, 28
positive airway pressure, 46
pulmonary function test, 58, 62
pulse oximetry, 28, 58, 63
pump failure, 27
quiet state of sleep, 17
REM sleep, 17

respiratory cycle, 20
restless leg syndrome, 43
rocking bed, 49
signs, 36
sleep arousal, 34
sleep latency, 37
sleep related breathing disorders, 19

smart CPAP, 52
snoring, 35
stages of sleep, 17
surgery, 48
symptoms, 36
tidal volume, 20
vasodilation, 37
water, 22

About the Author

Nicholas DiFilippo, D.O., FCCP, a Board Certified pulmonologist, has been practicing pulmonary medicine in the Chicago area some 30 years. Dr. DiFilippo has been "down in the trenches" treating patients with lung diseases. He has also authored a number of papers in the scientific journals including titles such as "Amiodarone and the Lung," "Pressure Support Ventilation," and "The Recurrence of Alveolitis in Interstitial Lung Disease." He has served as consultant in pulmonary medicine, medical staff president, chairman of a department of internal medicine, and director of pulmonary medicine. He is board certified by The American Board of Internal Medicine, in Internal Medicine and in Pulmonary Diseases. He is a Fellow of the American College of Chest Physicians (FCCP). Currently Dr. DiFilippo is associated with Internal Medicine and Pulmonary Diseases, Ltd., Oak Lawn, Illinois.

Made in the USA
Las Vegas, NV
27 May 2024

90445548R00039